CHOLESTEROL FREE COOKBOOK

Dr. Penny Watson

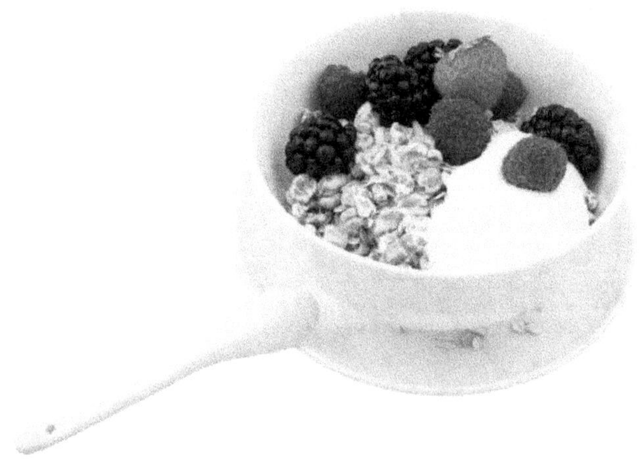

TABLE OF CONTENTS

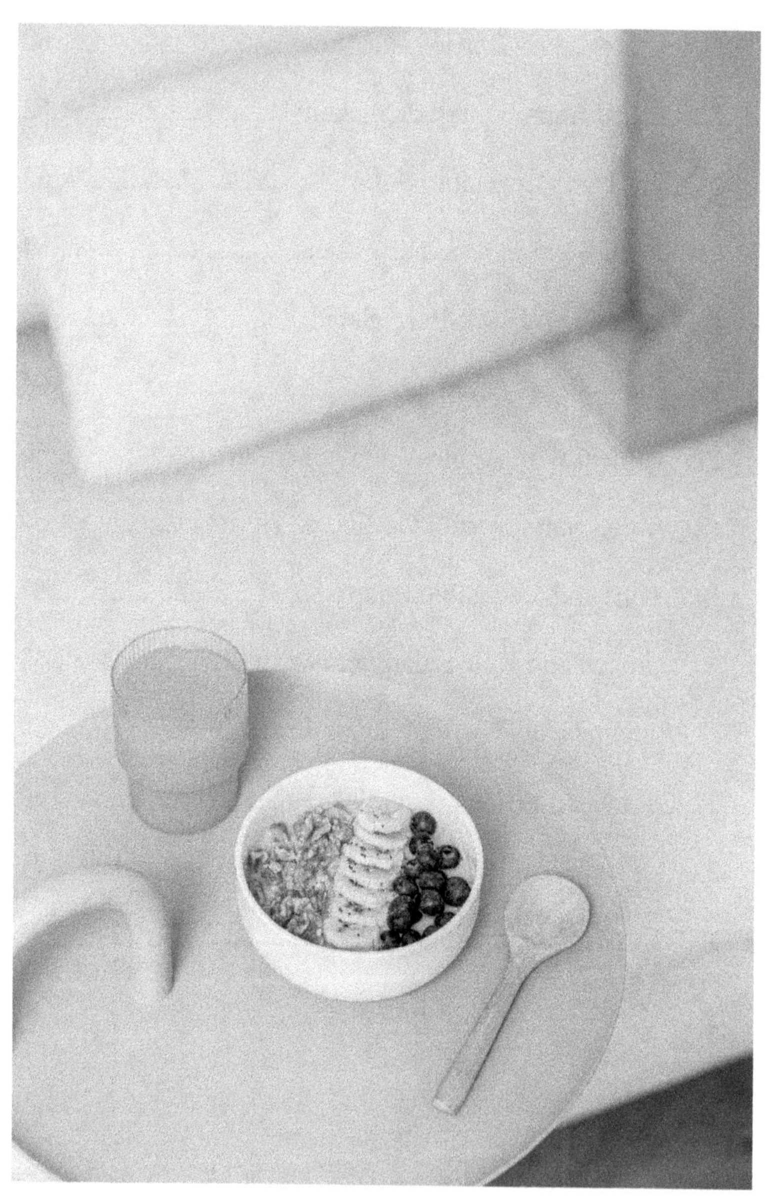

INTRODUCTION

Once upon a time in a bustling city, there lived a man named Sam. Concerned about his health, he embarked on a journey to regulate his cholesterol levels. He embraced a diet rich in whole grains, fresh fruits, and vegetables. Sam replaced red meat with lean proteins like fish and chicken, while nuts and olive oil became his allies. Regular exercise also found a place in his daily routine.

Over time, Sam's dedication bore fruit as his cholesterol levels balanced, energizing him to explore life's adventures with renewed vigor. With every heart-healthy meal, he rewrote his own story, proving that with the right diet, one could savor life's joys to the fullest.

Your body needs some cholesterol to work properly. But if you have too much in your blood, it can stick to the walls of your arteries and narrow or even block them. This puts you at risk for coronary artery disease and other heart diseases.

Cholesterol travels through the blood on proteins called lipoproteins. One type, LDL, is sometimes called the "bad" cholesterol. A high LDL level leads to a buildup of cholesterol in your arteries.

Another type, HDL, is sometimes called the "good" cholesterol. It carries cholesterol from other parts of your body back to your liver. Then your liver removes the cholesterol from your body.

What are the treatments for high cholesterol?

The treatments for high cholesterol are heart-healthy lifestyle changes and medicines. The lifestyle changes include healthy eating, weight management, and regular physical activity.

How can I lower cholesterol with diet?

Heart-healthy lifestyle changes include a diet to lower your cholesterol. The DASH eating plan is one example. Another is the Therapeutic Lifestyle Changes diet, which recommends that you

Choose healthier fats. You should limit both total fat and saturated fat. No more than 25 to 35% of your daily calories should come from dietary fats, and less than 7% of your daily calories should come from saturated fat. Depending upon how many calories you eat per day, here are the maximum amounts of fats that you should eat:

Saturated fat is a bad fat because it raises your LDL (bad cholesterol) level more than anything else in your diet. It is found in some meats, dairy products, chocolate, baked goods, and deep-fried and processed foods.

Trans fat is another bad fat; it can raise your LDL and lower you HDL (good cholesterol). Trans fat is mostly in foods made with hydrogenated oils and fats, such as stick margarine, crackers, and french fries.

Instead of these bad fats, try healthier fats, such as lean meat, nuts, and unsaturated oils like canola, olive, and safflower oils.

Limit foods with cholesterol. If you are trying to lower your cholesterol, you should have less than 200 mg a day of cholesterol. Cholesterol is in foods of animal origin, such as liver and other organ meats, egg yolks, shrimp, and whole milk dairy products.

Eat plenty of soluble fiber. Foods high in soluble fiber help prevent your digestive tract from absorbing cholesterol.

These foods include:

• Whole-grain cereals such as oatmeal and oat bran

• Fruits such as apples, bananas, oranges, pears, and prunes

• Legumes such as kidney beans, lentils, chick peas, black-eyed peas, and lima beans

Eat lots of fruits and vegetables

A diet rich in fruits and vegetables can increase important cholesterol-lowering compounds in your diet. These compounds, called plant stanols or sterols, work like soluble fiber.

Eat fish that are high in omega-3 fatty acids. These acids won't lower your LDL level, but they may help raise your HDL level.

They may also protect your heart from blood clots and inflammation and reduce your risk of heart attack. Fish that are a good source of omega-3 fatty acids include salmon, tuna (canned or fresh), and mackerel. Try to eat these fish two times a week.

Limit salt. You should try to limit the amount of sodium (salt) that you eat to no more than 2,300 milligrams (about 1 teaspoon of salt) a day.

That includes all the sodium you eat, whether it was added in cooking or at the table, or already present in food products. Limiting salt won't lower your cholesterol, but it can lower your risk of heart diseases by helping to lower your blood pressure.

You can reduce your sodium by instead choosing low-salt and "no added salt" foods and seasonings at the table or while cooking.

Limit alcohol. Alcohol adds extra calories, which can lead to weight gain. Being overweight can raise your LDL level and lower your HDL level. Too much alcohol can also increase your risk of heart diseases because it can raise your blood pressure and triglyceride level. One drink is a glass of wine, beer, or a small amount of hard liquor, and the recommendation is that:

- Men should have no more than two drinks containing alcohol a day
- Women should have no more than one drink containing alcohol a day

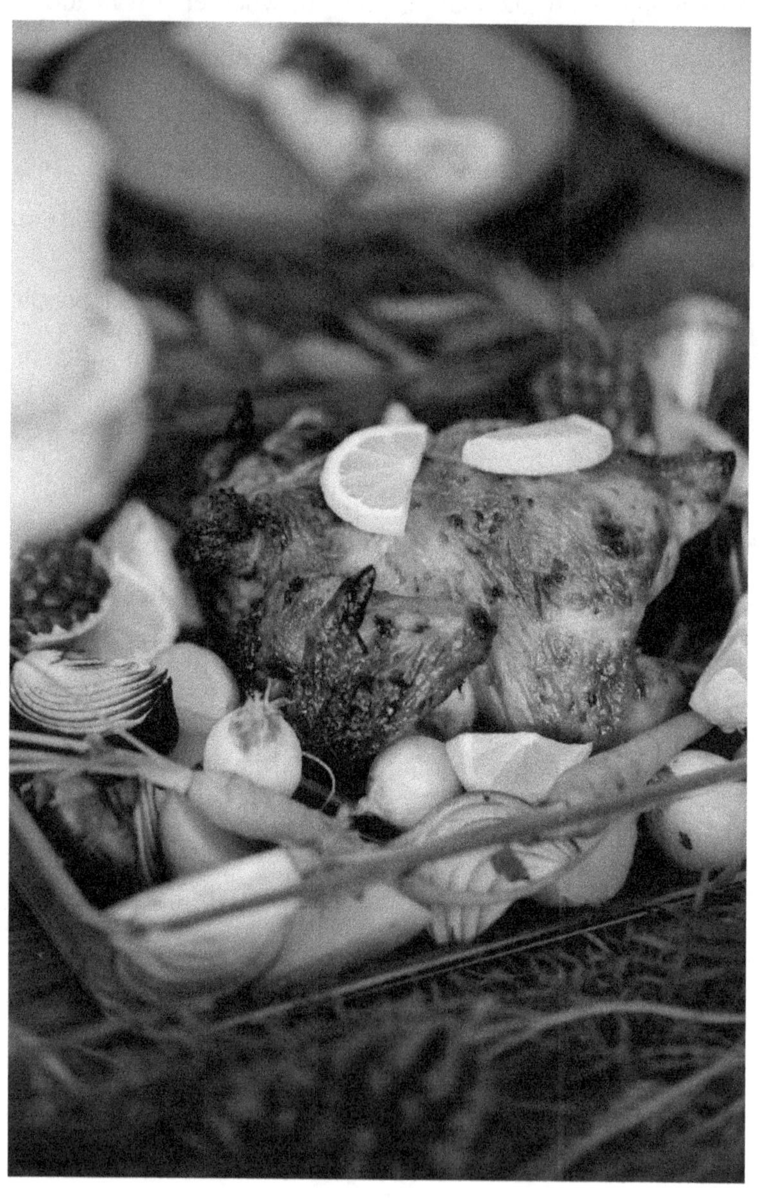

CHAPTER ONE

BEST DIET FOR CHOLESTEROL CONTROL (Scientific Proof)

If you're trying to implement healthier eating habits, it can be tough to figure out where to start. Maybe one of your friends has been trying to get you to cut added sugars for years now while another swears that going gluten-free changed her life. Thankfully, emerging research is here to make your choice easier.

A new study published in the Journal of the American College of Nutrition compared two of the most popular diets right now, the vegan diet and the Mediterranean diet, to see how they affected participants' weight as well as other risk factors for heart disease. The results? Sticking to a low-fat vegan diet is better for your health than going with the Mediterranean

The evidence is clear that a plant-based diet is a great way to manage weight and that all the side effects are good ones—from boosting heart health and improving cholesterol to lowering the risk for diabetes," corresponding author Hana

Kahleova, MD, PhD, MBA, Director of Clinical Research at the Physicians Committee for Responsible Medicine told Eat This, Not That! in an interview.

More specifically, the study found that the vegan diet can lower "bad" cholesterol levels known as LDL, improve insulin sensitivity, and lead to more weight loss. The Mediterranean diet's only win was that it led to an even greater blood pressure decrease than the low-fat vegan diet, though both diets yielded positive effects. It is also worth noting that the study did not require participants to count calories or track nutrients.

"We weren't surprised to see that people saw improvements on the plant-based diet," said Kahleova. "But, because the Mediterranean diet is often touted for weight loss, it was surprising to see that participants experienced very small changes—if any at all—when it came to their weight."

How is cholesterol measured?

Cholesterol is measured using a blood test called a 'lipid profile'.

This measures total cholesterol, HDL cholesterol and LDL cholesterol, as well as triglycerides — another type of fat in the blood. You will normally be asked to fast (not eat anything) and only drink water for about 10 hours before the test.

How often should I have my cholesterol tested?

Adults should have their blood lipids measured every 5 years, starting at 45 years. Aboriginal and Torres Strait Islander people should start lipid blood tests at 35, because on average heart and blood vessel disease — such as heart attacks and stroke — happen 10 to 20 years earlier in Indigenous people.

All Australians in these age groups are eligible for a regular 20-minute heart health check with their doctor. This checks your blood pressure, cholesterol and blood sugar levels. Your doctor can then assess your risk of having a heart attack or stroke in the next 5 years.

What are the risks linked to high cholesterol?

Too much LDL (bad) cholesterol in the blood can increase your risk of heart and blood vessel disease (cardiovascular disease).

The excess LDL cholesterol leads to fatty deposits called plaque forming in the artery walls. Over time, the plaque causes narrowing and hardening of the arteries (known as atherosclerosis).

This can lead to:

• **Angina** — when plaque builds up in the major arteries that supply your heart, known as the coronary arteries, they become narrower and are partially blocked, reducing blood flow and oxygen supply to the heart. This may cause shortness of breath and chest pain.

• **Heart attack** — if a plaque in a coronary artery bursts (ruptures), a clot may form and block the supply of blood to the heart, starving it of oxygen.

• **Stroke** — if the blood vessels that supply the brain become narrower or blocked by plaque, blood supply to the brain can be severely reduced or cut off, causing a stroke. Strokes can also be caused when a clot from another part of the body travels through the blood and lodges in an artery in the brain.

• **Peripheral vascular disease** — this usually affects the arteries that supply the legs and feet, causing leg pain when walking (known as intermittent claudication), and even pain when resting, when the circulation is more badly affected.

A high level of HDL cholesterol is good because HDL cholesterol helps remove other forms of cholesterol from the blood, taking them back to the liver — where they're removed from the blood and passed out of the body.

TOP FOODS TO IMPROVE YOUR NUMBERS

Diet can play an important role in lowering your cholesterol. Here are some foods to improve your cholesterol and protect your heart.

Can a bowl of oatmeal help lower your cholesterol? How about a handful of almonds?

A few simple tweaks to your diet — along with exercise and other heart-healthy habits — might help you lower your cholesterol.

Oatmeal, oat bran and high-fiber foods

Oatmeal contains soluble fiber, which reduces your low-density lipoprotein (LDL) cholesterol, the "bad" cholesterol. Soluble fiber is also found in such foods as kidney beans, Brussels sprouts, apples and pears.

Soluble fiber can reduce the absorption of cholesterol into your bloodstream. Five to ten grams or more of soluble fiber a day decreases your LDL cholesterol. One serving of a breakfast cereal with oatmeal or oat bran provides 3 to 4 grams of fiber.

If you add fruit, such as a banana or berries, you'll get even more fiber.

Fish and omega-3 fatty acids

Fatty fish has high levels of omega-3 fatty acids, which can reduce your triglycerides — a type of fat found in blood — as well as reduce your blood pressure and risk of developing blood clots. In people who have already had heart attacks, omega-3 fatty acids may reduce the risk of sudden death.

Omega-3 fatty acids don't affect LDL cholesterol levels. But because of those acids' other heart benefits, the American Heart Association recommends eating at least two servings of fish a week. Baking or grilling the fish avoids adding unhealthy fats.

The highest levels of omega-3 fatty acids are in:

- Mackerel
- Herring
- Tuna
- Salmon
- Trout

Foods such as walnuts, flaxseed and canola oil also have small amounts of omega-3 fatty acids.

Omega-3 and fish oil supplements are available. Talk to your doctor before taking any supplements.

Almonds and other nuts

Almonds and other tree nuts can improve blood cholesterol. A recent study concluded that a diet supplemented with walnuts can lower the risk of heart complications in people with history of a heart attack.

All nuts are high in calories, so a handful added to a salad or eaten as a snack will do.

Avocados

Avocados are a potent source of nutrients as well as monounsaturated fatty acids (MUFAs). Research suggests that adding an avocado a day to a heart-healthy diet can help improve LDL cholesterol levels in people who are overweight or obese.

People tend to be most familiar with avocados in guacamole, which usually is eaten with high-fat corn chips.

Try adding avocado slices to salads and sandwiches or eating them as a side dish. Also try guacamole with raw cut vegetables, such as cucumber slices.

Replacing saturated fats, such as those found in meats, with MUFAs are part of what makes the Mediterranean diet heart healthy.

Olive oil

Try using olive oil in place of other fats in your diet. You can saute vegetables in olive oil, add it to a marinade or mix it with vinegar as a salad dressing.

You can also use olive oil as a substitute for butter when basting meat or as a dip for bread.

Foods with added plant sterols or stanols

Sterols and stanols are substances found in plants that help block the absorption of cholesterol.

Foods that have been fortified with sterols or stanols are available.

Margarines and orange juice with added plant sterols can help reduce LDL cholesterol.

Adding 2 grams of sterol to your diet every day can lower your LDL cholesterol by 5 to 15 percent.

It's not clear whether food with plant sterols or stanols reduces your risk of heart attack or stroke — although experts assume that foods that reduce cholesterol do reduce the risk. Plant sterols or stanols don't appear to affect levels of triglycerides or of high-density lipoprotein (HDL) cholesterol, the "good" cholesterol.

Whey protein

Whey protein, which is found in dairy products, may account for many of the health benefits attributed to dairy. Studies have shown that whey protein given as a supplement lowers both LDL and total cholesterol as well as blood pressure. You can find whey protein powders in health food stores and some grocery stores.

Other changes to your diet

Getting the full benefit of these foods requires other changes to your diet and lifestyle.

One of the most beneficial changes is limiting the saturated and trans fats you eat.

Saturated fats — such as those in meat, butter, cheese and other full-fat dairy products — raise your total cholesterol. Decreasing your consumption of saturated fats to less than 7 percent of your total daily calorie intake can reduce your LDL cholesterol by 8 to 10 percent.

Trans fats, sometimes listed on food labels as "partially hydrogenated vegetable oil," are often used in margarines and store-bought cookies, crackers and cakes. Trans fats raise overall cholesterol levels.

The Food and Drug Administration has banned the use of partially hydrogenated vegetable oils by Jan. 1, 2021.

Foods that make up a low cholesterol diet can help reduce high levels

Changing what foods you eat can lower your cholesterol and improve the armada of fats floating through your bloodstream.

Adding foods that lower LDL, the harmful cholesterol-carrying particle that contributes to artery-clogging atherosclerosis, is the best way to achieve a low cholesterol diet.

Add these foods to lower LDL cholesterol

Different foods lower cholesterol in various ways. Some deliver soluble fiber, which binds cholesterol and its precursors in the digestive system and drags them out of the body before they get into circulation. Some give you polyunsaturated fats, which directly lower LDL. And some contain plant sterols and stanols, which block the body from absorbing cholesterol.

1. Oats. An easy first step to lowering your cholesterol is having a bowl of oatmeal or cold oat-based cereal like Cheerios for breakfast. It gives you 1 to 2 grams of soluble fiber. Add a banana or some strawberries for another half-gram. Current nutrition guidelines recommend getting 20 to 35 grams of fiber a day, with at least 5 to 10 grams coming from soluble fiber. (The average American gets about half that amount.)

2. Barley and other whole grains. Like oats and oat bran, barley and other whole grains can help lower the risk of heart disease, mainly via the soluble fiber they deliver.

3. Beans. Beans are especially rich in soluble fiber. They also take a while for the body to digest, meaning you feel full for longer after a meal. That's one reason beans are a useful food for folks trying to lose weight. With so many choices — from navy and kidney beans to lentils, garbanzos, black-eyed peas, and beyond — and so many ways to prepare them, beans are a very versatile food.

4. Eggplant and okra. These two low-calorie vegetables are good sources of soluble fiber.

5. Nuts. A bushel of studies shows that eating almonds, walnuts, peanuts, and other nuts is good for the heart. Eating 2 ounces of nuts a day can slightly lower LDL, on the order of 5%. Nuts have additional nutrients that protect the heart in other ways.

6. Vegetable oils. Using liquid vegetable oils such as canola, sunflower, safflower, and others in place of butter, lard, or shortening when cooking or at the table helps lower LDL.

7. Apples, grapes, strawberries, citrus fruits. These fruits are rich in pectin, a type of soluble fiber that lowers LDL.

8. Foods fortified with sterols and stanols. Sterols and stanols extracted from plants gum up the body's ability to absorb cholesterol from food.

Companies are adding them to foods ranging from margarine and granola bars to orange juice and chocolate. They're also available as supplements. Getting 2 grams of plant sterols or stanols a day can lower LDL cholesterol by about 10%.

9. Soy. Eating soybeans and foods made from them, like tofu and soy milk, was once touted as a powerful way to lower cholesterol. Analyses show that the effect is more modest — consuming 25 grams of soy protein a day (10 ounces of tofu or 2 1/2 cups of soy milk) can lower LDL by 5% to 6%.

10. Fatty fish. Eating fish two or three times a week can lower LDL in two ways: by replacing meat, which has LDL-boosting saturated fats, and by delivering LDL-lowering omega-3 fats. Omega-3s reduce triglycerides in the bloodstream and also protect the heart by helping prevent the onset of abnormal heart rhythms.

11. Fiber supplements. Supplements offer the least appealing way to get soluble fiber.

Two teaspoons a day of psyllium, which is found in Metamucil and other bulk-forming laxatives, provide about 4 grams of soluble fiber.

Putting together a low cholesterol diet

When it comes to investing money, experts recommend creating a portfolio of diverse investments instead of putting all your eggs in one basket.

The same holds true for eating your way to lower cholesterol. Adding several foods to lower cholesterol in different ways should work better than focusing on one or two.

A largely vegetarian "dietary portfolio of cholesterol-lowering foods" substantially lowers LDL, triglycerides, and blood pressure. The key dietary components are plenty of fruits and vegetables, whole grains instead of highly refined ones, and protein mostly from plants.

Add margarine enriched with plant sterols; oats, barley, psyllium, okra, and eggplant, all rich in soluble fiber; soy protein; and whole almonds.

Of course, shifting to a cholesterol-lowering diet takes more attention than popping a daily statin. It means expanding the variety of foods you usually put in your shopping cart and getting used to new textures and flavors.

But it's a "natural" way to lower cholesterol, and it avoids the risk of muscle problems and other side effects that plague some people who take statins.

Just as important, a diet that is heavy on fruits, vegetables, beans, and nuts is good for the body in ways beyond lowering cholesterol. It keeps blood pressure in check.

It helps arteries stay flexible and responsive. It's good for bones and digestive health, for vision and mental health.

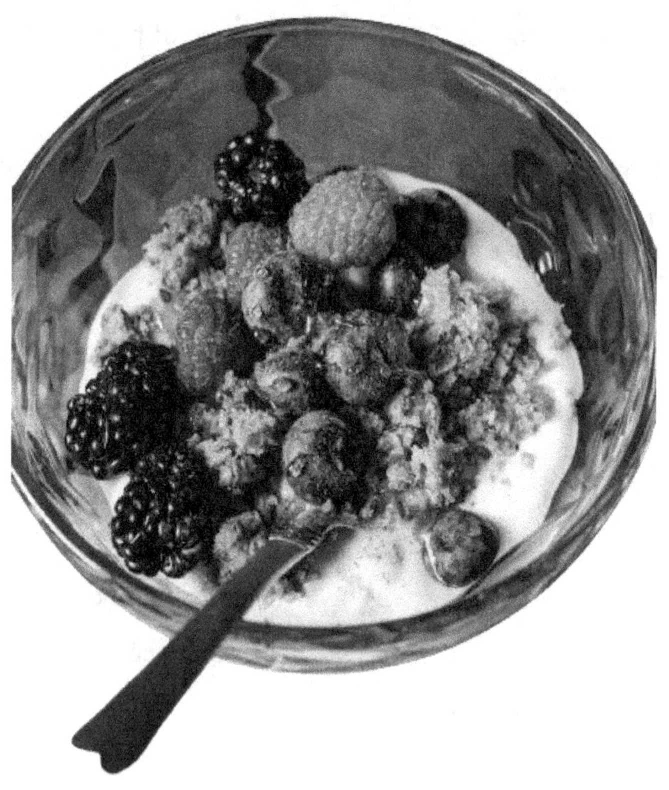

CHAPTER TWO

HEALTHY EATING TIPS TO LOWER CHOLESTEROL

As well as sticking to a varied and healthy diet, try these tips to help you manage your cholesterol:

• The Heart Foundation recommends that people follow a heart-healthy eating pattern, which is built on eating mostly plant-based foods. Eating more plant-based foods like vegetables, legumes, fruit, wholegrains, nuts and seeds is good for heart health.

Include legumes (or pulses such as chickpeas, lentils, split peas), beans (such as haricot beans, kidney beans, baked beans, bean mixes) in at least two meals a week. Check food labels and choose the lowest sodium (salt) products.

Beans make a great alternative to meat in tacos, or snack on hummus with vegetable sticks. You can also add legumes to soups, pasta sauces, curries and stews.

Use tofu or lentils instead of meat in stir fries or curries.

• Choose wholegrain breads, cereals, pasta, rice and noodles.

• Snack on plain, unsalted nuts and fresh fruit (ideally two serves of fruit every day).

• Use avocado, nut butters, tahini or spreads made from healthy unsaturated fats (such as canola, sunflower or extra virgin olive oil) instead of those made with saturated fat (such as butter, coconut oil and cream).

• Use healthy oils for cooking – some include canola, sunflower, soybean, olive (extra virgin is a good choice), sesame and peanut oils.

• For people at high risk of heart disease, the Heart Foundation recommends people eat 2-3 grams of plant sterol-enriched foods every day (for example, plant sterol-enriched margarine, yoghurt, milk and cereals).

• Enjoy fish two to three times a week (150 grams fresh or 100g tinned).

• Most people don't need to limit the number of eggs they eat each week. However, a maximum of seven eggs each week is recommended for people with high cholesterol, type 2 diabetes and heart disease.

Select lean meat (meat trimmed of fat, and poultry without skin) and limit unprocessed red meat to less than 350g per week.

• Choose unflavoured milk, yoghurt and cheese. People with high cholesterol or heart disease should opt for reduced fat options. Check the labels to make sure there's no added sugar. Non-dairy milks and yoghurts are ok too; opt for versions that have no added sugar and have had calcium added.

• Limit or avoid processed meats including sausages and deli meats (such as ham, bacon and salami).

You can also speak to an Accredited Practising Dietitian for specific advice.

Check out the Heart Foundation website for a range of simple, delicious recipes including vegetarian recipes and those that include plant-based proteins such as lentils, chickpeas and beans:

Dietary fibre

If you are trying to lower your cholesterol, aim to eat foods that are high in dietary fibre (particularly soluble fibre), because they can reduce the amount of LDL (bad) cholesterol in your blood.

You can increase your fibre intake by eating:

- fruit

- vegetables

- legumes (such as chickpeas, lentils, soybeans and bean mixes)

- wholegrains (for example, oats and barley)

- nuts and seeds.

Dietary fats

Following a healthy, balanced diet that is low in saturated fats and trans-fats can help to lower your cholesterol.

Aim to replace foods that contain unhealthy, saturated and trans-fats with foods that contain healthy fats.

Unhealthy fats

Foods high in (unhealthy) saturated fats include:

- processed or deli-style meats (such as ham, bacon and salami)

- deep fried fast foods

- processed foods (such as biscuits and pastries)

- takeaway foods (such as hamburgers and pizza)

- fat on meat and skin on chicken

- ghee, lard and copha

- coconut oil

- palm oil (often called vegetable oil in products) cream and ice cream

- butter.

- Foods high in (unhealthy) trans fats include:

- deep fried foods

- baked goods (such as pies, pastries, cakes and biscuits)

- takeaway foods

- butter

- foods that list 'hydrogenated oils' or 'partially hydrogenated vegetable oils' on the ingredients list.

Healthy fats

Foods high in (healthy) polyunsaturated fats include:

- soybean, sunflower, safflower, canola oil and margarine spreads made from these oils

- pine nuts, walnuts and brazil nuts.

- fish
- tahini (sesame seed spread)
- linseed (flaxseed) and chia seeds
- Foods high in (healthy) monounsaturated fats include:
- cooking oils made from plants or seeds, including: olive, canola, peanut, sunflower, soybean, sesame and safflower
- avocados
- olives
- unsalted nuts such as almonds, cashews and peanuts.

Triglycerides in your blood

In addition to cholesterol, your blood also contains a type of fat called triglycerides, which are stored in your body's fat deposits.

Hormones release triglycerides to make energy between meals.

When you eat, your body converts any extra energy (kilojoules) it doesn't need right away into triglycerides.

Like cholesterol, your body needs triglycerides to work properly. However, there is evidence to suggest that some people with high triglycerides are at increased risk of heart disease and stroke.

If you regularly eat more energy than you need, you may have high triglycerides.

Lowering triglycerides

Some ways to reduce triglyceride levels include:

• stick to a healthy diet by following a heart-healthy eating pattern and limiting unhealthy fats, salt and added sugar

• opt for water, tea and coffee (without adding sugar) as heart-healthy drinks, instead of sugar-sweetened drinks (such as soft drinks, cordial, energy drinks and sports drinks)

• include foods with healthy omega-3 fats (for example, fish such as salmon, sardines and tuna)

• reduce or limit your alcohol intake

• maintain a healthy weight and reduce fat around your middle.

Treatment for high cholesterol

Making lifestyle changes, especially changing some of the foods you eat, and regular physical activity, are very important to help reduce high LDL (bad) cholesterol.

• Move more. Regular physical activity is one of the best things you can do for your heart health. Increasing your physical activity from as little as 10 minutes a day to the Australian government's recommended 30 to 45 minutes a day, five or more days of the week, can help manage your cholesterol levels and reduce your risk of heart disease.

• Quitting smoking reduces the risk of heart disease and can help reduce cholesterol levels. The most effective way to stop smoking is with a combination of stop-smoking medicines (like nicotine replacement therapy) and support from a service like Quitline (Tel: 13 78 48). Speaking to your GP is also a great first step.

• Drinking alcohol doesn't have any health benefits. Alcohol contributes unnecessary kilojoules (energy) and is of low nutritional value. Alcohol is not a necessary or recommended part of a heart-healthy eating pattern. If you do drink, to reduce your risk of alcohol-related harm, healthy women and men should drink no more than 10 standard drinks a week and no more than four standard drinks on any one day.

• You may also need to take cholesterol-lowering medicines (such as statins) to help manage your cholesterol and reduce your risk of having a heart attack or stroke. Talk to your doctor about finding the most appropriate treatment for you.

7 DAY MEAL PLAN TO LOWER BLOOD CHOLESTEROL LEVEL

Certainly, here's a 7-day meal plan to help lower blood cholesterol levels. This plan focuses on reducing saturated fats and incorporating foods that promote heart health:

Day 1:

Breakfast:

- Oatmeal topped with fresh berries and a sprinkle of flaxseeds.
- A glass of unsweetened almond milk.

Lunch:

- Grilled chicken breast with a side of steamed broccoli and quinoa.
- A mixed greens salad with vinaigrette dressing.

Snack:

- Greek yogurt with honey and a handful of almonds.

Dinner:

- Baked salmon with a lemon-dill sauce.
- Roasted Brussels sprouts and a small serving of brown rice.

Day 2:

Breakfast:

- Whole-grain toast with mashed avocado and a poached egg.
- A serving of sliced grapefruit.

Lunch:

- Lentil soup with a side of mixed greens salad (include heart-healthy nuts and seeds).

Snack:

- Sliced cucumber with hummus.

Dinner:

- Grilled shrimp with asparagus and whole-grain pasta.
- A side of steamed spinach.

Day 3:

Breakfast:

- A green smoothie made with spinach, banana, unsweetened almond milk, and chia seeds.

Lunch:

- Chickpea salad with mixed vegetables, dressed with olive oil and balsamic vinegar.

Snack:

- Carrot sticks with a tablespoon of almond butter.

Dinner:

- Baked chicken breast with roasted sweet potatoes and broccoli.

Day 4:

Breakfast:

- Greek yogurt parfait with granola and fresh berries.
- A glass of green tea.

Lunch:

- Quinoa and black bean stuffed bell peppers.

Snack:

- A handful of walnuts and dried apricots.

Dinner:

- Baked cod with a side of sautéed spinach and quinoa.

Day 5:

Breakfast:

- Scrambled eggs with spinach and diced tomatoes.
- A slice of whole-grain toast.

Lunch:

- Tuna salad made with Greek yogurt and loaded with vegetables, served in a whole-grain wrap.

Snack:

- Sliced bell peppers with guacamole.

Dinner:

- Grilled tofu with a side of stir-fried broccoli, bell peppers, and brown rice.

Day 6:

Breakfast:

- Overnight oats with almond milk, sliced banana, and a sprinkle of cinnamon.

Lunch:

- Spinach and feta stuffed chicken breast with steamed asparagus.

Snack:

- A piece of dark chocolate (at least 70% cocoa).

Dinner:

- Lentil and vegetable curry served with brown rice.

Day 7:

Breakfast:

- Whole-grain waffles topped with Greek yogurt and mixed berries.

Lunch:

- Grilled vegetables and quinoa salad with a tahini dressing.

Snack:

- A boiled egg.

Dinner:

- Baked salmon with a side of sautéed kale and wild rice.

Remember to drink plenty of water throughout the day and maintain portion control. This meal plan, along with regular exercise, can help you in your efforts to lower blood cholesterol levels. Consulting with a healthcare professional or registered dietitian is advisable for personalized guidance and to ensure your specific dietary needs are met.

CHAPTER THREE

CHOLESTEROL FREE DIET RECIPES

1. Chicken with Bell Pepper & Hominy Stir-Fry

INGREDIENTS

- 2 teaspoons canola oil
- 1 ¼ pounds boneless, skinless chicken breast, trimmed and cut into 1-inch pieces
- 3 teaspoons ground cumin, divided
- ½ teaspoon kosher salt, divided
- ½ cup finely chopped fresh cilantro
- 2 medium red bell peppers, chopped
- 2 cups sliced carrots
- 1 ½ cups chopped red onion
- 3 tablespoons water
- 2 cups rinsed canned hominy
- 2 cloves garlic, minced
- 1 (4 ounce) can diced green chiles
- 2 tablespoons lime juice
- 1 firm ripe avocado, diced

DIRECTIONS

- **Step 1**

Heat oil in a large nonstick skillet over medium-high heat.

Add chicken and sprinkle with 1 teaspoon cumin and 1/4 teaspoon salt. Cook, stirring occasionally, until the chicken is just cooked through, 5 to 7 minutes.

Transfer to a bowl and toss with cilantro. Cover to keep warm.

- **Step 2**

Add bell peppers, carrots, onion, water and the remaining 1/4 teaspoon salt to the pan. Cook, stirring often, until the vegetables are crisp-tender, about 5 minutes.

Stir in hominy, garlic and the remaining 2 teaspoons cumin; cook, stirring, for 1 minute. Stir in green chiles and lime juice and cook for 1-minute more.

- **Step 3**

Serve the chicken over the hominy mixture, topped with avocado.

2. Ratatouille with White Beans & Polenta

INGREDIENTS

- 5 tablespoons extra-virgin olive oil, divided
- 1 large onion, coarsely chopped
- 1 medium red bell pepper, chopped
- 4 cloves garlic, minced
- 1 small eggplant, cut into 1/2-inch chunks
- ½ teaspoon kosher salt, divided
- 2 medium zucchini, halved lengthwise and sliced
- 1 (15 ounce) can no-salt-added white beans, rinsed
- 1 pint cherry or grape tomatoes, halved
- ¼ cup slivered sun-dried tomatoes
- 1 teaspoon Italian seasoning
- 1 tablespoon capers, rinsed and chopped
- ½ teaspoon ground pepper
- 1 16- to 18-ounce tube prepared polenta (see Tip), sliced into 8 rounds
- ¼ cup toasted pine nuts

DIRECTIONS

- **Step 1**

Heat 1 tablespoon oil in a large pot over medium heat. Add onion and bell peppers, sprinkle with 1/8 teaspoon salt; cook, stirring occasionally, until the vegetables soften, 5 to 7 minutes. Add garlic and; cook, stirring, until fragrant, about 1 minute more. Transfer the vegetables to a large bowl.

- **Step 2**

Add 1 tablespoon oil to the pot. Add eggplant, sprinkle with 1/4 teaspoon salt and cook, stirring frequently, until browned in places, 4 to 6 minutes. Transfer to the bowl with the vegetables.

- **Step 3**

Add another 2 tablespoons oil to the pot. Add zucchini, sprinkle with the remaining 1/8 teaspoon salt and cook, stirring frequently, until browned in places, 3 to 5 minutes. Add beans, cherry (or grape) tomatoes, sun-dried tomatoes, Italian seasoning, pepper and the reserved vegetables; stir to combine.

Reduce heat to medium-low, cover and cook, stirring occasionally, until the vegetables are tender, 8 to 10 minutes.

• **Step 4**

Meanwhile, heat remaining 1 tablespoon oil in a large nonstick skillet over medium heat. Add polenta rounds and cook until golden brown on the bottom, about 5 minutes. Turn each slice and cook until browned on the second side, about 5 minutes more.

• **Step 5**

Stir capers into the ratatouille. Serve the polenta and the ratatouille topped with pine nuts.

Tips: Look for convenient tubes of precooked polenta in the pasta aisle or near refrigerated tofu at the supermarket.

3. Mixed Greens with Lentils & Sliced Apple

INGREDIENTS

- 1 ½ cups mixed salad greens
- ½ cup cooked lentils
- 1 apple, cored and sliced, divided

- 1 ½ tablespoons crumbled feta cheese

- 1 tablespoon red-wine vinegar

- 2 teaspoons extra-virgin olive oil

Directions

Top greens with lentils, about half the apple slices and the feta. Drizzle with vinegar and oil. Serve with the remaining apple slices on the side.

4. Bean & Butternut Tacos with Green Salsa

INGREDIENTS

Salsa

- 8 ounces tomatillos

- 2 cloves garlic, unpeeled

- 1 jalapeño pepper

- ¼ cup sliced white onion

- ½ ripe avocado, diced

- 3 tablespoons chopped fresh cilantro

- ¼ teaspoon salt

- Freshly ground pepper to taste

Tacos

- 4 cups diced (1/2-inch) peeled butternut squash
- 3-4 small dried red chiles
- 2 cloves garlic, unpeeled, smashed and left whole
- 1 tablespoon extra-virgin olive oil
- 3/4 teaspoon dried oregano, preferably Mexican, divided
- ½ teaspoon salt, divided
- 1/4 teaspoon cumin seeds, plus 1/2 teaspoon ground toasted cumin seeds (see Tip), divided
- 2 cups cooked pinto beans, drained (see Tip)
- ½ teaspoon chili powder
- Freshly ground pepper to taste
- 8 6-inch corn tortillas
- ½ cup fresh cilantro leaves
- ½ cup finely shredded and chopped red or green cabbage
- 8 teaspoons crumbled queso fresco (see Note), or feta cheese

DIRECTIONS

- **Step 1**

To prepare salsa: Bring a pot of water to a boil. Remove husks from tomatillos and rinse well. Cook the tomatillos in the boiling water until soft, 5 to 8 minutes. Drain and set aside.

- **Step 2**

Toast garlic cloves, jalapeno and onion in a dry medium skillet over medium heat, turning occasionally, until browned, fragrant and soft, 5 to 7 minutes.

- **Step 3**

When cool enough to handle, peel the garlic. Remove the jalapeno stem and remove seeds if desired.

Combine the tomatillos, garlic, jalapeno, onion and avocado in a blender or food processor. Process until smooth. Stir in cilantro, salt and pepper. Set aside for topping the tacos.

- **Step 4**

To prepare tacos: Preheat oven to 400 degrees F.

- **Step 5**

Put squash in a medium bowl and, using kitchen shears, finely snip chiles to taste into small pieces (seeds and all) into the bowl.

Add garlic, oil, 1/2 teaspoon oregano, 1/4 teaspoon salt and whole cumin seeds; toss to coat. Arrange on a baking sheet in a single layer. Bake until soft and beginning to brown, 20 to 25 minutes. Peel and finely chop the garlic when cool enough to handle; stir into the squash.

- **Step 6**

Meanwhile, combine beans in a small saucepan with the remaining 1/4 teaspoon oregano and 1/4 teaspoon salt, ground cumin, chili powder and pepper. Heat over medium-low heat for about 10 minutes.

- **Step 7**

Warm tortillas one at a time in a dry large cast-iron (or similar heavy) skillet over medium heat until soft and pliable.

Wrap in a clean towel to keep warm as you go. Spoon 1/4 cup of the warm beans into each tortilla; divide the roasted squash evenly among the tacos and top each with cilantro, cabbage, 1/2 cup of the salsa and cheese. (Refrigerate the remaining 1/2 cup salsa for up to 2 days.)

TIPS

Make Ahead Tip: The salsa can be prepared ahead (Step 1-3). Cover and refrigerate for up to 2 days.

Tip: Toast cumin seeds in a small skillet over medium heat, stirring occasionally, until very fragrant, 2 to 5 minutes.

Let cool. Grind into a powder in a spice mill or blender.

5. Pan-Seared Steak with Crispy Herbs & Escarole

INGREDIENTS

- 1-pound sirloin steak, about 1/2 inch thick
- ½ teaspoon salt, divided
- ½ teaspoon ground pepper, divided
- 2 tablespoons grapeseed oil or canola oil
- 4 cloves garlic, crushed
- 5 sprigs fresh thyme
- 3 sprigs fresh sage

-   1 sprig fresh rosemary

-   16 cups chopped escarole (about 1 pound)

DIRECTIONS

- **Step 1**

Sprinkle steak with 1/4 teaspoon each salt and pepper. Heat a large cast-iron skillet over medium-high heat.

Add the steak and cook until charred on one side, about 3 minutes.

Turn the steak over and add oil, garlic, thyme, sage and rosemary. Cook, stirring the herbs occasionally, until an instant-read thermometer inserted in the thickest part of the steak reaches 125 degrees F for medium-rare, 3 to 4 minutes. Transfer the steak to a plate and top with the garlic and herbs. Tent with foil.

- **Step 2**

Add escarole and the remaining 1/4 teaspoon each salt and pepper to the pan. Cook, stirring often, until the escarole starts to wilt, about 2 minutes. Thinly slice the steak and serve with the escarole and crispy herbs

6. Spaghetti Squash with Roasted Tomatoes, Beans & Almond Pesto

INGREDIENTS

Almond Pesto

- 2 cups fresh basil leaves
- 1 cup fresh parsley leaves
- ½ cup grated Parmesan cheese
- ⅓ cup whole raw almonds
- 1 clove garlic
- 1 ½ tablespoons red-wine vinegar
- ¼ teaspoon kosher salt
- ¼ teaspoon ground pepper
- ¼ cup extra-virgin olive oil
- ¼ cup water
- Spaghetti Squash & Vegetables
- 1 3-pound spaghetti squash
- ¼ cup water
- 2 pints grape tomatoes, halved
- 1 tablespoon extra-virgin olive oil
- ¼ teaspoon kosher salt

-   ¼ teaspoon ground pepper

-   1 cup canned cannellini beans, rinsed

DIRECTIONS

• **Step 1**

To prepare pesto: Pulse basil, parsley, Parmesan, almonds, garlic, vinegar and 1/4 teaspoon each salt and pepper in a food processor until coarsely chopped, scraping down the sides. With the motor running, add 1/4 cup oil; process until well combined.

• **Step 2**

Add water to the pesto in the food processor; pulse to combine.

• **Step 3**

To prepare squash & vegetables: Preheat oven to 400 degrees F. Line a rimmed baking sheet with foil.

• **Step 4**

Halve squash lengthwise and scoop out the seeds. Place cut-side down in a microwave-safe dish and add water.

Microwave on High until the flesh can be easily scraped with a fork, about 15 minutes.

• **Step 5**

Meanwhile, toss tomatoes with oil, salt and pepper in a large bowl. Transfer to the prepared baking sheet. Roast until soft and wrinkled, 10 to 12 minutes. Remove from the oven. Add beans and stir to combine.

• **Step 6**

Scrape the squash flesh into the bowl and divide among 4 plates. Top each portion with some of the tomato-bean mixture and about 3 tablespoons pesto sauce.

TIPS

To make ahead: Refrigerate pesto (Step 1) for up to 5 days.

Tips: Turn leftovers into a pesto-turkey sandwich for lunch: Spread 1 1/2 Tbsp. leftover pesto on 2 slices toasted whole-wheat bread. Top with 3 oz. sliced deli turkey, 2 lettuce leaves and 2 tomato slices.

7. Creamy Chicken, Brussels Sprouts & Mushrooms One-Pot Pasta

Ingredients

- 8 ounces whole-wheat linguine or spaghetti
- 1-pound boneless, skinless chicken thighs
- 4 cups sliced mushrooms
- 2 cups sliced Brussels sprouts
- 1 medium onion, chopped
- 4 cloves garlic, thinly sliced
- 2 tablespoons Boursin cheese
- 1 ¼ teaspoons dried thyme
- ¾ teaspoon dried rosemary
- ¾ teaspoon salt
- 4 cups water
- 2 tablespoons chopped fresh chives

DIRECTIONS

- **Step 1**

Combine pasta, chicken, mushrooms, Brussels sprouts, onion, garlic, Boursin cheese, thyme, rosemary and salt in a large pot. Stir in water.

Bring to a boil over high heat. Boil, stirring frequently, until the pasta is cooked and the water has almost evaporated, 10 to 12 minutes.

Remove from heat and let stand, stirring occasionally, for 5 minutes.

Serve sprinkled with chives.

8. Chicken Sausage and Peppers

INGREDIENTS

- Nonstick cooking spray
- 4 medium red, yellow, orange, and/or green sweet peppers, cut into 1-inch pieces
- 1 large sweet onion, cut into thin wedges
- 2 cups grape tomatoes
- 1 tablespoon olive oil
- 1 tablespoon balsamic vinegar
- 1 12 ounce pkg. Italian-flavor cooked chicken sausage, bias-sliced into thirds
- 1 tablespoon snipped fresh oregano
- Toasted baguette slices (optional)

DIRECTIONS

- **Step 1**

Preheat oven to 425°F. Coat a 15x10-inch baking pan with cooking spray.

In the prepared pan combine peppers, onion, and tomatoes. Drizzle with oil and vinegar; toss gently to coat. Roast 30 minutes.

- **Step 2**

Push vegetables to one side, exposing about one-fourth of the pan. Place sausage in pan. Roast 10 to 15 minutes more or until vegetables are tender and sausage is heated through. Top with oregano. If desired, serve with toasted baguette slices.

9. Chicken Chili with Sweet Potatoes

INGREDIENTS

- 2 tablespoons extra-virgin olive oil
- 1 large onion, chopped
- 3 cloves garlic, minced
- 2 cups cubed sweet potato (1/2-inch)

- 1 medium green bell pepper, chopped

- 2 tablespoons chili powder

- 2 teaspoons ground cumin

- 1 teaspoon dried oregano

- 1 15-ounce can low-sodium cannellini beans, rinsed

- 2 cups low-sodium chicken broth or homemade chicken stock

- 1 cup frozen corn

- 2 cups cubed cooked chicken (1/2-inch; about 10 ounces)

- ¾ teaspoon salt

- ¼ teaspoon ground pepper

- Sour cream, avocado and/or cilantro for garnish

DIRECTIONS

• **Step 1**

Heat oil in a large pot over medium-high heat. Add onion, garlic, sweet potato and bell pepper; cook, stirring occasionally, until the vegetables are slightly softened, 5 to 6 minutes. Stir in chili powder, cumin and oregano and cook, stirring, until fragrant, 1 minute.

- **Step 2**

Add beans and broth (or stock) and bring to a boil. Reduce heat, partially cover and simmer gently for 15 minutes.

- **Step 3**

Increase heat to medium-high and stir in corn; cook 1 minute. Add chicken and cook until heated through, 1 to 2 minutes more. Remove from heat. Stir in salt and pepper. Serve topped with sour cream, avocado and/or cilantro, if desired.

10. Oatmeal with Chia and Berries:

Ingredients:

- 1/2 cup rolled oats
- 1 tablespoon chia seeds
- 1/2 cup mixed berries (strawberries, blueberries, raspberries)
- 1 cup almond milk

Method:

1. Combine oats and chia seeds in a bowl.
2. Add almond milk and mix well.

3. Let it sit in the refrigerator overnight.

4. In the morning, top with mixed berries.

11. Oatmeal with Berries and Nuts:

Ingredients:

- 1/2 cup old-fashioned oats

- 1 cup unsweetened almond milk

- 1/2 cup fresh berries (e.g., blueberries, strawberries)

- 1 tablespoon chopped nuts (e.g., almonds, walnuts)

- 1 teaspoon honey (optional)

Method:

1. In a saucepan, bring almond milk to a simmer.

2. Stir in oats and cook until creamy, about 5 minutes.

3. Top with berries, nuts, and a drizzle of honey if desired.

12. Grilled Lemon Garlic Chicken:

Ingredients:

- 4 boneless, skinless chicken breasts

- 2 cloves garlic, minced

- Zest and juice of 1 lemon

- 1 tablespoon olive oil

- Fresh herbs (e.g., rosemary, thyme), chopped

- Salt and pepper to taste

Method:

1. In a bowl, combine minced garlic, lemon zest, lemon juice, olive oil, herbs, salt, and pepper.
2. Marinate chicken breasts in the mixture for at least 30 minutes.
3. Grill the chicken until fully cooked, about 6-8 minutes per side.

13. Lentil and Vegetable Soup

Ingredients:

- 1 cup dried lentils, rinsed and drained

- 4 cups vegetable broth

- 1 onion, chopped

- 2 carrots, diced

- 2 celery stalks, diced

- 2 cloves garlic, minced

- 1 teaspoon dried thyme

- Salt and pepper to taste

Method:

1. In a large pot, sauté onion, carrots, and celery in olive oil until softened.
2. Add garlic, lentils, thyme, and vegetable broth. Bring to a boil.
3. Reduce heat, cover, and simmer for about 30 minutes until lentils are tender.

14. Baked Salmon with Dill Sauce:

Ingredients:

- 4 salmon fillets
- 2 tablespoons chopped fresh dill
- 2 tablespoons plain Greek yogurt
- 1 tablespoon Dijon mustard
- 1 teaspoon lemon juice
- Salt and pepper to taste

Method:

1. Preheat the oven to 375°F (190°C).
2. Place salmon fillets on a baking sheet.
3. In a bowl, mix dill, Greek yogurt, Dijon mustard, lemon juice, salt, and pepper.

4. Spread the sauce evenly over the salmon.

5. Bake for about 15-20 minutes until salmon flakes easily with a fork.

15. Quinoa and Black Bean Salad:

Ingredients:

- 1 cup quinoa, cooked and cooled

- 1 can (15 oz) black beans, rinsed and drained

- 1 cup cherry tomatoes, halved

- 1/2 cup diced red bell pepper

- 1/4 cup chopped fresh cilantro

- 2 tablespoons olive oil

- 1 tablespoon lime juice

- Salt and pepper to taste

Method:

1. In a large bowl, combine quinoa, black beans, cherry tomatoes, red bell pepper, and cilantro.

2. In a separate bowl, whisk together olive oil, lime juice, salt, and pepper.

3. Toss the quinoa salad with the dressing until well combined.

16. Baked Sweet Potatoes:

Ingredients:

- 4 medium sweet potatoes
- 1 tablespoon olive oil
- 1 teaspoon smoked paprika
- Salt and pepper to taste

Method:

1. Preheat the oven to 400°F (200°C).
2. Scrub sweet potatoes and pierce them with a fork.
3. Rub olive oil, smoked paprika, salt, and pepper over the sweet potatoes.
4. Place them on a baking sheet and bake for 45-60 minutes until tender.

17. Oatmeal with Apples and Cinnamon:

Ingredients:

- 1 cup rolled oats
- 1 apple, diced
- 1/2 teaspoon ground cinnamon
- 1 tablespoon honey (optional)

Method:

1. Cook rolled oats according to package instructions.
2. Top with diced apples, sprinkle with cinnamon, and drizzle with honey if desired.

18. Grilled Salmon with Garlic and Herbs

Ingredients:

- 4 salmon fillets (4-6 oz each)
- 2 cloves garlic, minced
- 2 tablespoons fresh chopped herbs (such as rosemary, thyme, and parsley)
- 2 tablespoons olive oil
- Salt and pepper to taste

Method:

1. Mix minced garlic, herbs, olive oil, salt, and pepper.
2. Brush the mixture onto salmon fillets, grill for 4-5 minutes per side.

19. Lentil and Vegetable Soup

Ingredients:

- 1 cup dried green lentils

- 1 onion, chopped

- 2 carrots, diced

- 2 celery stalks, diced

- 2 cloves garlic, minced

- 8 cups low-sodium vegetable broth

- 1 teaspoon cumin

- 1 teaspoon paprika

- Salt and pepper to taste

Method:

1. In a large pot, sauté onions, carrots, celery, and garlic until softened.
2. Add lentils, broth, and spices.
3. Simmer for 30-40 minutes until lentils are tender.

20. Spinach and Kale Salad with Walnuts

Ingredients:

- 4 cups baby spinach

- 2 cups kale, chopped

- 1/2 cup walnuts, toasted

- 2 tablespoons olive oil

- 2 tablespoons balsamic vinegar

- 1/4 cup crumbled feta cheese

- Salt and pepper to taste

Method:

1. Toss spinach, kale, and walnuts.

2. Drizzle with olive oil and balsamic vinegar.

3. Sprinkle with feta, salt, and pepper.

21. Chickpea and Vegetable Stir-Fry:

Ingredients:

- 1 can (15 oz) chickpeas, drained and rinsed

- 2 cups broccoli florets

- 1 red bell pepper, sliced

- 2 cloves garlic, minced

- 2 tablespoons low-sodium soy sauce

- 1 tablespoon sesame oil

- 1/2 teaspoon ginger, grated

Method:

1. Heat sesame oil in a pan, sauté garlic and ginger.

2. Add chickpeas, broccoli, and bell pepper.

3. Stir in soy sauce and cook until vegetables arc tender.

22. Quinoa and Black Bean Salad

Ingredients:

- 1 cup quinoa
- 1 can (15 oz) black beans, drained and rinsed
- 1 cup corn kernels (fresh or frozen)
- 1 red onion, finely chopped
- 1/4 cup cilantro, chopped
- Juice of 2 limes
- 2 tablespoons olive oil
- Salt and pepper to taste

Method:

1. Cook quinoa and let it cool.
2. In a large bowl, combine quinoa, black beans, corn, red onion, and cilantro.
3. Drizzle with lime juice and olive oil. Season with salt and pepper.

23. Baked Sweet Potatoes with Avocado Salsa

Ingredients:

- 4 medium sweet potatoes
- 2 ripe avocados, diced
- 1 tomato, diced
- 1/4 cup red onion, finely chopped
- Juice of 2 limes
- 1/4 cup fresh cilantro, chopped
- Salt and pepper to taste

Method:

1. Bake sweet potatoes until tender.
2. In a bowl, combine diced avocados, tomato, red onion, lime juice, cilantro, salt, and pepper.
3. Serve salsa over baked sweet potatoes.

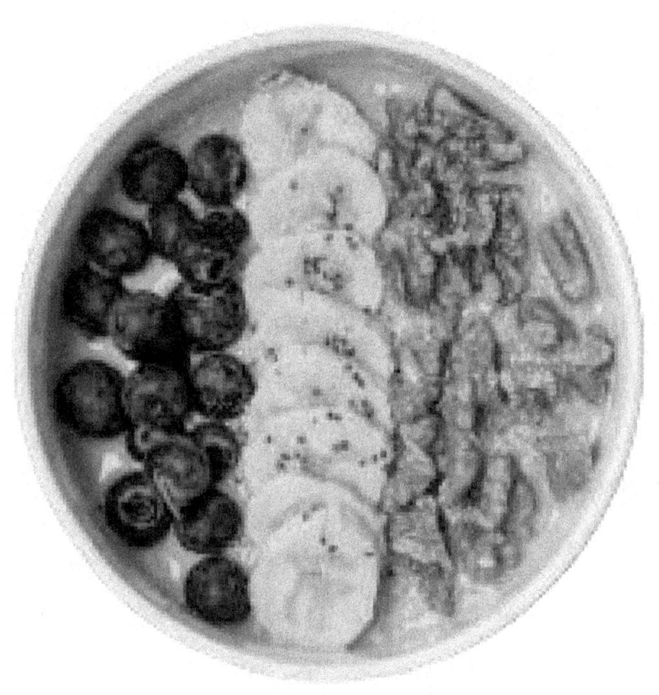

CONCLUSION

High cholesterol levels are a major risk factor for heart disease.

Thankfully, you can lower this risk by incorporating certain foods into your diet.

Upping your intake of these foods will put you on the path to a balanced diet and keep your heart healthy.

You can also practice techniques like mindful eating to make sure you're enjoying your meal and getting full without overdoing it.

In conclusion, this cholesterol-free cookbook offers a flavorful journey toward better heart health.

We have explored a variety of delicious recipes that not only tantalize the taste buds but also promote overall well-being by helping to lower cholesterol levels.

By choosing ingredients wisely and preparing dishes thoughtfully, we've demonstrated that maintaining a heart-healthy diet can be both enjoyable and satisfying.

Throughout this cookbook, we've emphasized the use of wholesome, nutrient-rich ingredients, such as oats, salmon, lentils, and fresh vegetables.

These recipes showcase the power of food as medicine, highlighting the positive impact it can have on our cardiovascular health.

As we close the pages of this cookbook, let us remember that our choices in the kitchen can play a significant role in our heart health.

By incorporating these cholesterol-lowering recipes into our daily lives, we can take proactive steps toward reducing the risk of heart disease and ensuring a vibrant, cholesterol-free future.

Here's to nourishing our hearts and savoring every bite along the way!